Cosmetic Surgery

Do I Really Need It?

A Guide to Plastic Surgery

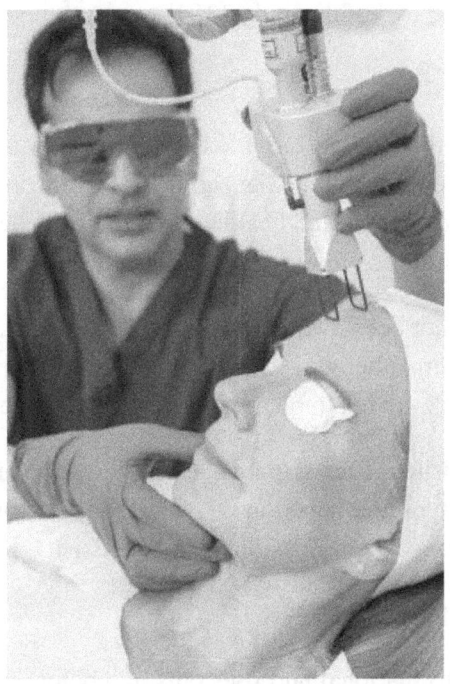

Healthy learning Series

Dueep Jyot Singh

Mendon Cottage Books

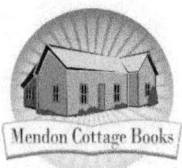

JD-Biz Publishing

Disclaimer

The information is this book is provided for informational purposes only. It is not intended to be used and medical advice or a substitute for proper medical treatment by a qualified health care provider. The information is believed to be accurate as presented based on research by the author.

The contents have not been evaluated by the U.S. Food and Drug Administration or any other Government or Health Organization and the contents in this book are not to be used to treat cure or prevent disease.

The author or publisher is not responsible for the use or safety of any diet, procedure or treatment mentioned in this book. The author or publisher is not responsible for errors or omissions that may exist.

Warning

The Book is for informational purposes only and before taking on any diet, treatment or medical procedure, it is recommended to consult with your primary health care provider.

Our books are available at

1. Amazon.com

2. Barnes and Noble

3. Itunes

4. Kobo

5. Smashwords

6. Google Play Books

Table of Contents

Introduction

You are going to be surprised to know that the trend for plastic surgery, – also known as cosmetic surgery and reconstructive aesthetic surgery – is turning out to be a multibillion-dollar business worldwide.

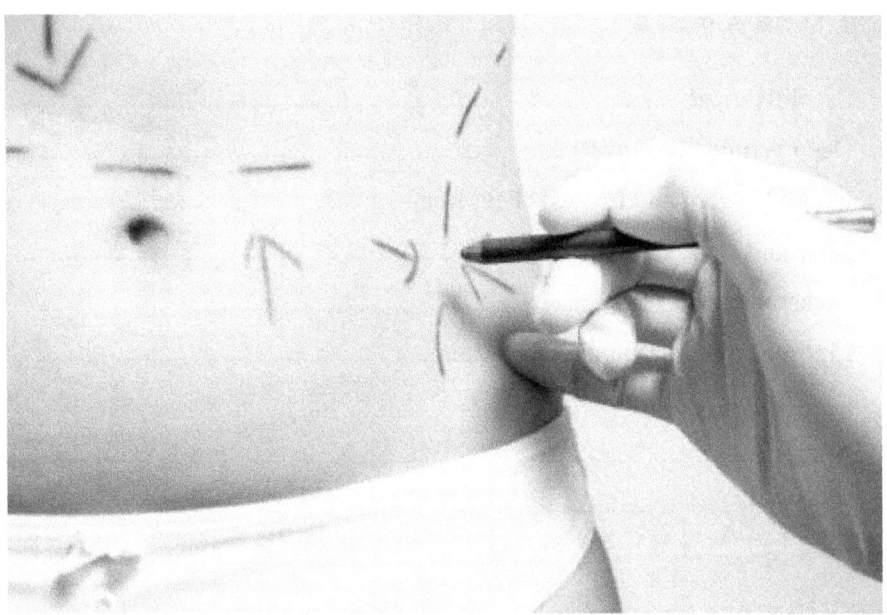

There are supposedly more cosmetic surgeons in some cities, than there are practicing general practitioners, or even medical specialists? Why is this so?

This book is going to tell you all about cosmetic surgery, and why people have some preconceived notions about it. Also, it is going to tell you all about surgical methods, which are practiced by reconstructive aesthetic surgeons – the new terminology for cosmetic surgeons – in order to make you look more youthful, beautiful, or just plain different.

Many people know about one of the scariest socialites in the USA. She has spent $4 million in the past 10 years and more so that she can look more like a cat instead of a human being. Her justification for spending all this money, in spoiling a perfectly once beautiful face and making it look grotesque and weird, is that her multimillionaire husband loves big cats, and she wants to keep him interested in her. So that is why she is looking for that perpetual feline look.

Any woman who can go to these limits in order to keep the fickle interest of Mr. Multi-Bank Accounts is definitely suffering from an infinity complex or she does not have anything constructive to do with her time. But this seems to please her. It also gets her plenty of attention because I think she enjoys the gawking audience staring at her and wondering how one could prefer to look so ugly. Especially when some of her surgical procedures made certain that she did not need a costume on Halloween in order to scare the kiddies.

So, here we come to these points – do you really need plastic surgery? What are the psychological aspects of this surgery on the psyche of a human being? What is the difference between cosmetic and plastic surgery?

This book is going to tell you all about reconstructive plastic surgery, and its steadily gaining importance in the life and times of beauty obsessed human beings.

Cosmetic surgery has become such a booming business, just because of good PR. The demand for some people to look like a popular concept of beauty is being encouraged by media people, as well as the surgeons themselves, so that more and more people go in for cosmetic and reconstructive surgery.

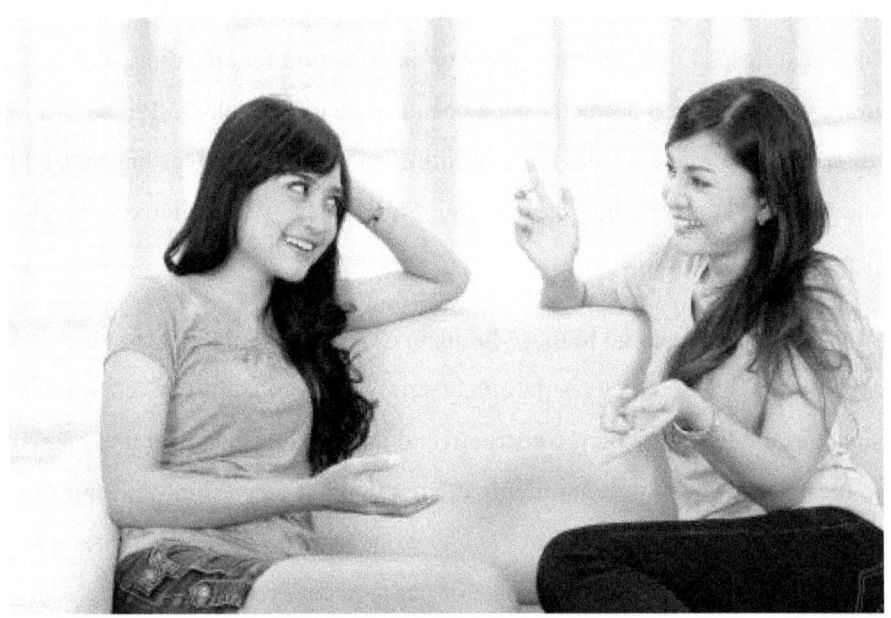

Did you know that there is the new cosmetic surgeon in town?

Historical Aspect

Reconstructive plastic surgery is not a new concept. Believe it or not, it has been around for more than 5000 years, especially in the east, when rhinoplasty was practiced by experienced surgeons on warriors, who had lost their noses in battle. A flap of flesh was taken from a not so visible part of the body and shaped into a nose.

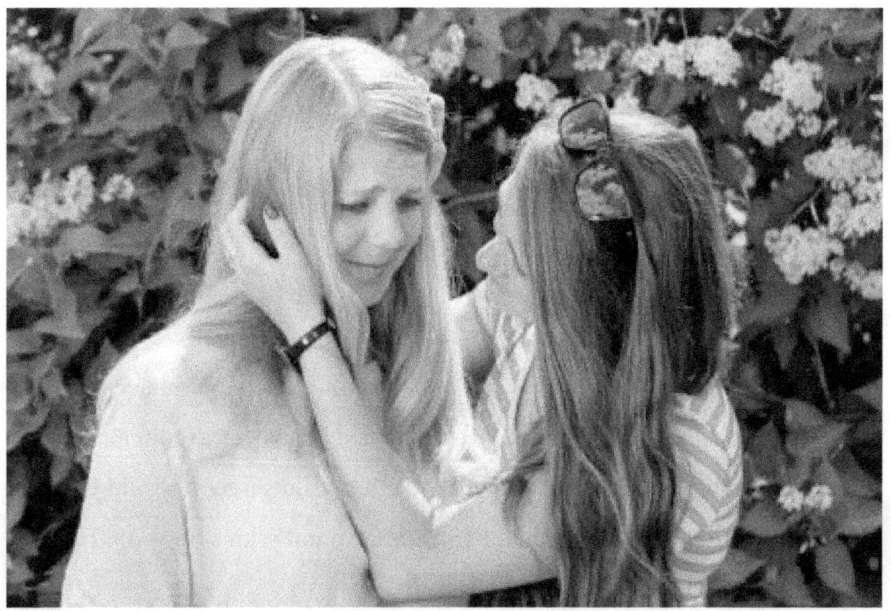

Just let me see what they did to your nose…

There are many reconstructive surgical procedures written in these ancient compendiums. But somehow they did not manage to reach the West, in ancient times and definitely not in the medieval times, even though the

Crusaders returning back from the battlefields of Constantinople and Jerusalem brought with them some useful and timeworn surgical knowledge and procedures as practiced by the Eastern surgeons.

Nevertheless cosmetic surgery in the West, in medieval times, especially in the dark ages was not a thing to be considered. That was when apothecaries and barbers used their own barbaric ways in order to either heal or kill.

It is a well-known fact that anybody suffering from a wound would have been bled with leeches or cupped with sharp knives. I remember reading a 17th-century history book, in which the heroine calls an Eastern servant trying to save his wounded master's life a monster and a savage.

The servant had just opened up the battle wound to get rid of the suppuration. The heroine would rather have had her man die of fever, gangrene and worse rather than trying any timeworn cure, which smacked of witchcraft!

If that person had been wounded in the 20th century, he would have been filled up with antibiotics. His wound has healed because it would have been treated in a hygienic manner. And after that a plastic surgeon would use his skill and experience to cover that disfiguring wound with skin taken from another part of the body.

However, nowadays, the concept of cosmetic surgery is more of changing and altering the shape of your visible organs, in order to look more youthful and more charming keeping in accordance with the modern perception of beauty.

Plastic surgery has nothing to do with plastic. It just means to mould and shape or form something. The word plastic has originated from the Greek word *plasto* which means "to sculpt".

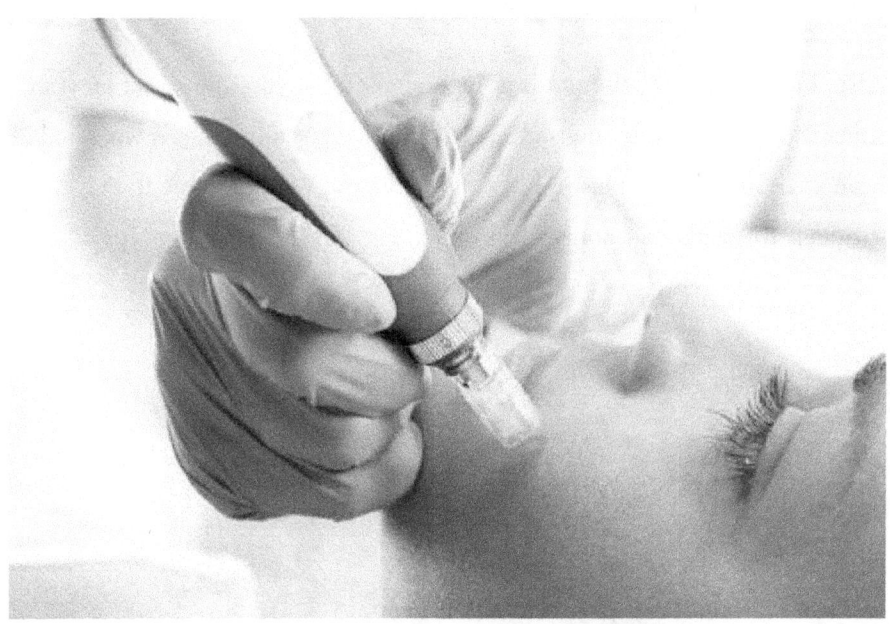

In the natural process of aging, the skin is going to lose its elasticity due to the atrophy of collagen fibers, and it is going to start to wrinkle. Some Cosmetic surgery procedures keep the wrinkles at bay, and you are going to learn more about them further on.

Also after pregnancy, the breasts start to sag, and the muscles of the stomach becomes "floppy." That is because the tissue of this area had to do an extended growth spurt in order to carry the baby for nine months. That is why, after the child has been delivered, women look at that flabby muscle and tissue growth and subconsciously associate it with unattractiveness.

Believe it or not, the tissue is going to regain its natural elasticity, with exercise, but most of us hate exercise in any form. We would rather submit to a surgeon's knife and get rid of it all in one go.

Also, overexposure to the sun is going to have a dehydrating effect on your skin. The dehydrated tissue is going to wrinkle up easily. This is what makes beauty companies and plastic surgeons so happy. Women come to these surgeons for facelifts, tummy tucks and the rest of the works.

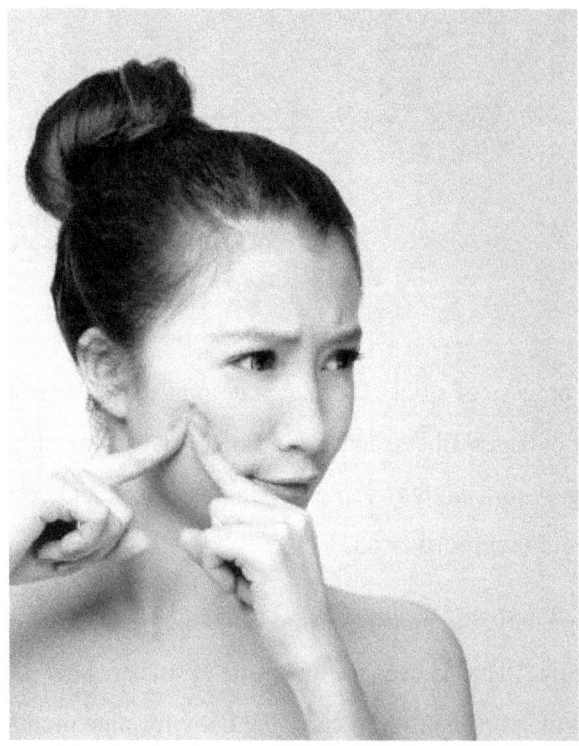

There is this little mark here…

Duration of Surgery

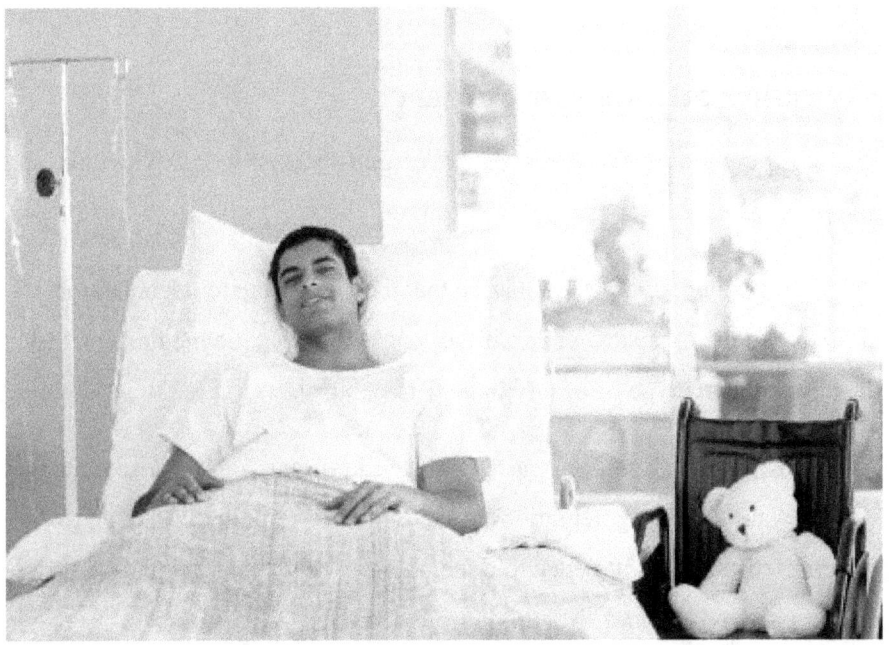

Surgical procedures of any kind need to be done under the close supervision of an experienced surgeon.

The surgical duration of cosmetic surgery or procedure is definitely not like going to a beauty parlor and getting ready for the Big Day. There are many things which are going to be taken into account by the surgeon.

These are going to include the age and the health of the prospective patient. He is also going to take into consideration the texture of the skin and the general psychological makeup of the patient.

Some people have such sensitive skin, that they are going to take more time for these scars to heal. You cannot be hundred percent sure about the scars and also whether you will begin to start looking like Ingrid Bergman, or The Latest Miss Universe.

Psychological Aspect of Surgery

Why consider the psychological aspect of a cosmetic surgery? Now this is one point which only a psychologist can tell you.

There are many people, who imagine that they are going to become more attractive to the opposite gender, if they look like what the media considers the popular stereotype of beauty in the 21st century.

That is why, apart from rhinoplasty – cosmetic surgery on the nose – many women want to get augmentations done to their bosom. I have a friend who is a cosmetic surgeon, he once told me, rather wryly, "many times women come to me and ask me, "Make Me Look like Her." And show me a picture of a seductive movie star half their age who is being touted as the latest, hottest sex kitten, if you would pardon my language."

When I asked him what he did under the circumstances, he just shrugged his shoulders. He told me that these women felt inadequate in some manner, because they had never been what they think is attractive. Since childhood, there has been someone criticizing their looks and giving them an inferiority complex.

One is sorry to say, but this is something inborn. The ideal idea of a beautiful woman in many parts of the world today is one of a particular skin tone, hair color, and eye color. This idea is being encouraged by the beauty industry, as well as publishers of escapist fiction, where you have idiotic novels about blonde and busty blue-eyed females managing to get the billionaire hero, while the slim, trim, brunette/redhead has to take a back seat.

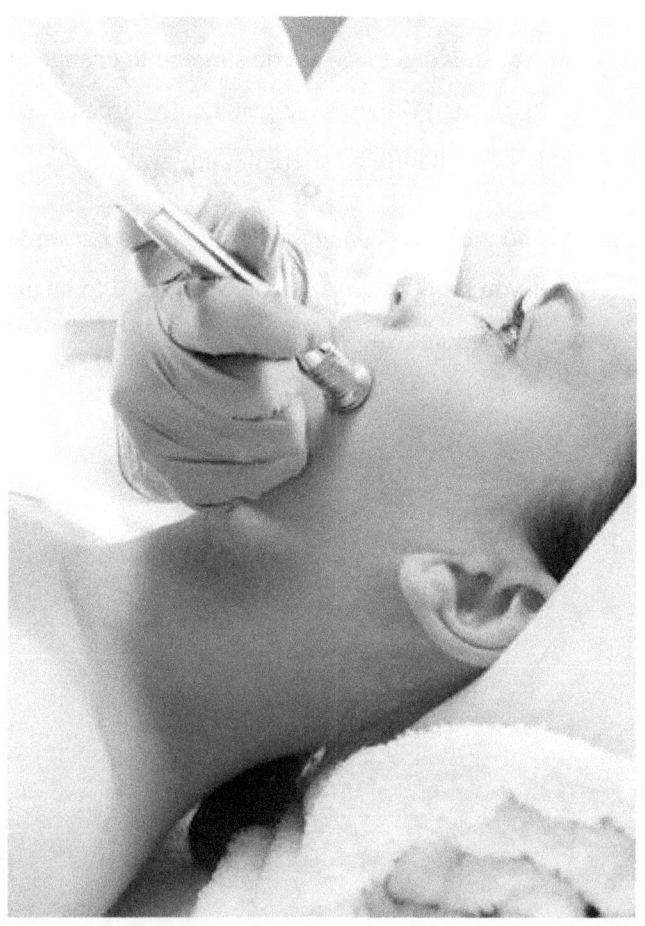

And so, with such stupid stories coming out from publishing houses in the millions, is it a wonder that a perfectly normal human being may begin to subconsciously want to look like someone else?

These women would never accept the fact that they had their own personal genetic makeup, cheekbones, features and skin texture. Shakira and Cindy Crawford's genes were not those of an ordinary woman, let us say, Fiona MacLean, Astrid Jorgenson, Mandy Liu, or, Deborah Rubenstein.

These women had their different racial genetic makeup given to them by their ancestors. So they could get a cosmetic surgeon to change the shapes of their noses, chins, lips, but if they were genetically large boned or tiny boned, their body shape could not be altered in any way.

Remember, there is no individual upon the earth, who is a completely hopeless case. What you think is ugly, can be considered to be the zenith of attractiveness and beauty somewhere else.

Reasons for Cosmetic Surgery

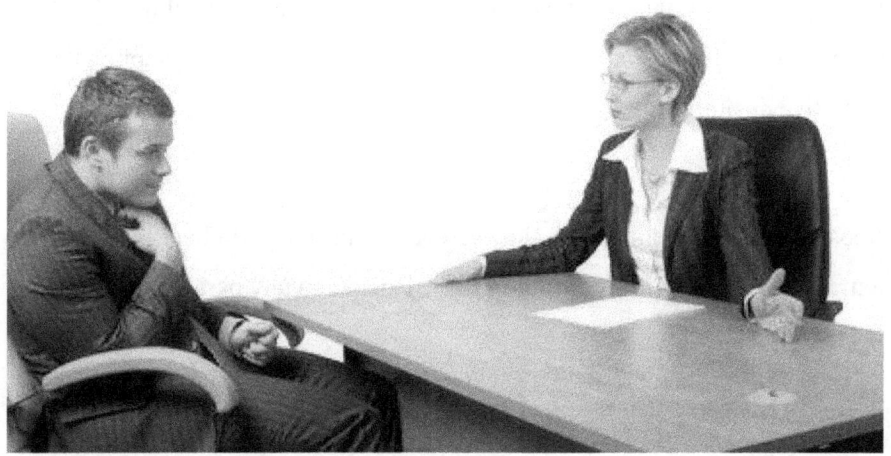

Apart from the very important reason of looking young for professional, and personal purposes, people going for cosmetic surgeries for social reasons too.

You are going to be surprised to know that a number of men come in cosmetic surgery. That is because they see their jobs going to people younger than they are. This insecurity makes them try surgery so that they can look younger.

Women forget that looks are a very superficial thing really, but when they begin to imagine that there has been bizarre partners are looking at youthful

---

and pretty girls, they begin to look at cosmetic surgery as an ego boosting alternative and also as a psychological support.

Social Aspects

When did this craze to change one's appearance in order to confirm with the social preconceived notion of what is beautiful and attractive start? Well, nobody is very certain about when people decided that skeletal females and even males with zero fat content would be considered to be the epitome of attractive desirability.

And that is why more and more women and men have begun to look at liposuction as a way in which they can get rid of that extra beer belly, the extra fat around their thighs or any fatty deposits in any part of their bodies.

This is definitely not a healthy trend. You may ask why. Man is naturally designed to have lots of fat in his body, in order to keep the system working properly. The fat content, under the skin was also a natural insulation for people, millenniums ago, when the skin was subjected to the raw and harsh elements of nature.

Man did not have hair covering his body like the majority of the beasts surrounding him. That is why he had to make do with the fat layer to keep him warm.

Even today in many parts of the world, the idea of good health and beauty is an obese and full figure. However, this trend began to change after the First World War, when starvation was the norm instead of the exception. And that is why the fashion designers had to make clothes for people who did not have enough of food during the deprivation age of war and the Depression following it.

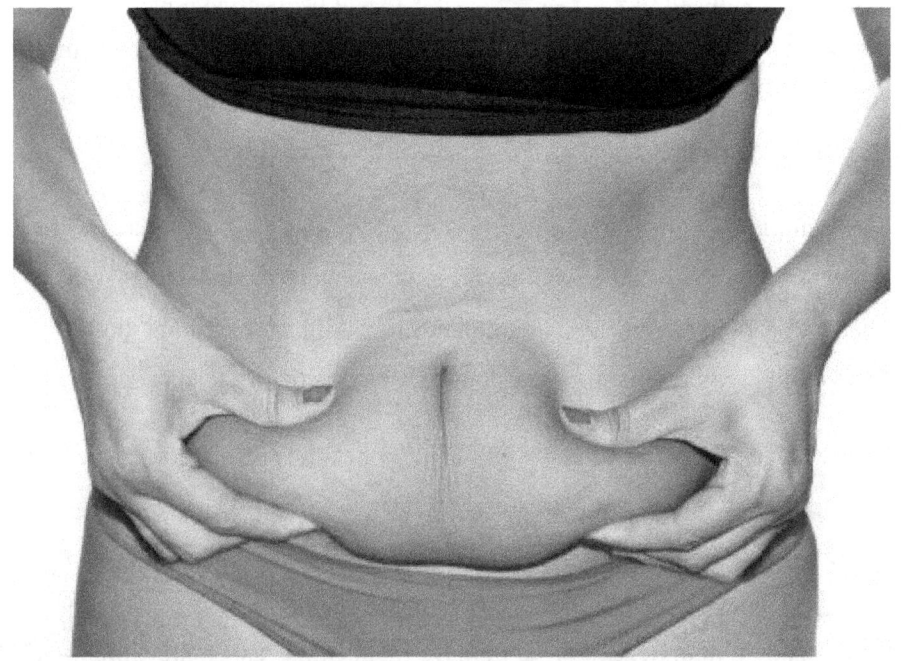

And so the rake thin, slim, and the Androgynous look came into existence. This also brought along with it, eating disorders in the 50s and 60s, because many people who had begun to find plentiful sources of food, after the war years of the 40s still could not manage to accept the fact that they could eat enough to grow fat.

Subconsciously, according to them, this was definitely not a proper thing. And that is why eating disorders and rake thin looks flourished.

Then in the 50s – 60s, another trend started when the concept of beauty began to be dictated by Hollywood, with women with overblown figures were considered to be "goddesses." Around this time, two supposed doctors came up with an idea that they could alter the figures of women to meet with the popular concept of 44 – 24 – 44. They began using silicon inserts under the bosom to boost up the chest area, so that one could be the ideal example of the *I must I must, develop my bust, the bigger the better, the tighter the sweater, the better the boys will like it* stream of thought.

These implants were done surgically. The aftermaths and the failures were many, but of course nobody bother telling the eager young ladies that the chances of infection and also the implants, breaking and harming the body were quite capable of being hazardous to their health, in the long run.

This was, of course, on par with 18th-century beauties painting their faces with lead paint in order to get the socially desirable and acceptable, white/pale and fragile complexion. And they died of lead poisoning. In the same manner Spanish beauties used to put drops of belladonna or Deadly Nightshade in their eyes in order to make them shine. They ended up blind.

Since then, plastic surgery or more properly called reconstructive aesthetic surgery is the surgery used to make a person look better. We know that in the eternal search for youth and beauty, people resort to many ways and means in order to look forever young and beautiful.

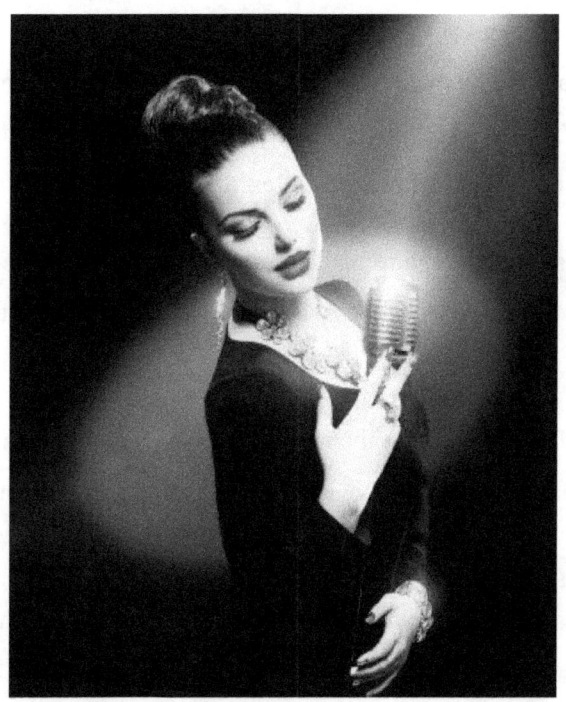

Also, the mind is conditioned to consider someone beautiful, because people have been saying so since day one. Now let me give you one example. When I was a kid, we used to live in an area, where we were a minority of fair complexioned, tall, and robust children. Our friends were short, stocky in physique, and dark in complexion.

We thought them beautiful, because they had such grace in their movements, just like little gazelles and beauty in their dark and dusky features and faces. And their mothers thought us "beautiful", – even though we were as gawky and awkward as galumphing baby giraffes – and definitely did not hesitate in showing their preferences, in the presence of their own kids.

We would have been cordially hated by one and all, until our friends noticed that we just hated to be the center of attention, especially in the Club, when all the mothers made a beeline for us to pull our cheeks and exclaim on our oh so desirable "red and white"[1] complexion.

It was embarrassing enough to make us children go right in the midday sun, and get baked as brown as berries, so that we got rid of that hated fair complexion.[2]

So this idea of beauty is all in the mind. And the beauty industry is feeding off it by encouraging one to have a Grecian profile, a Nordic bust, and so on.

When you know you have your own special magic, a boon inherited from your own personal glorious gene line, why would you want to look like someone else?

Nevertheless, because for all of us, the grass is always greener on the other side of the fence, and we are definitely not happy with what nature has given us, well, let us begin with facelifts.

But before that, I want to give you one last piece of advice – if you think that your happiness depends upon getting some feature changed, and you are immediately going to gain self-confidence, self-respect, and a boost to the Ego, I would suggest you talk to your cosmetic surgeon first.

---

[1] Their interpretation of pale sickly looking melanin challenged skin....

[2] The mothers definitely could not understand why anybody would want to destroy a perfectly charming, desirable, and white complexion on purpose. That was to prevent them from pulling our cheeks, kissing us wholesale, and exclaiming on how "beautiful" we were! Pfui, as Nero Wolfe would say, like a cat sneezing!

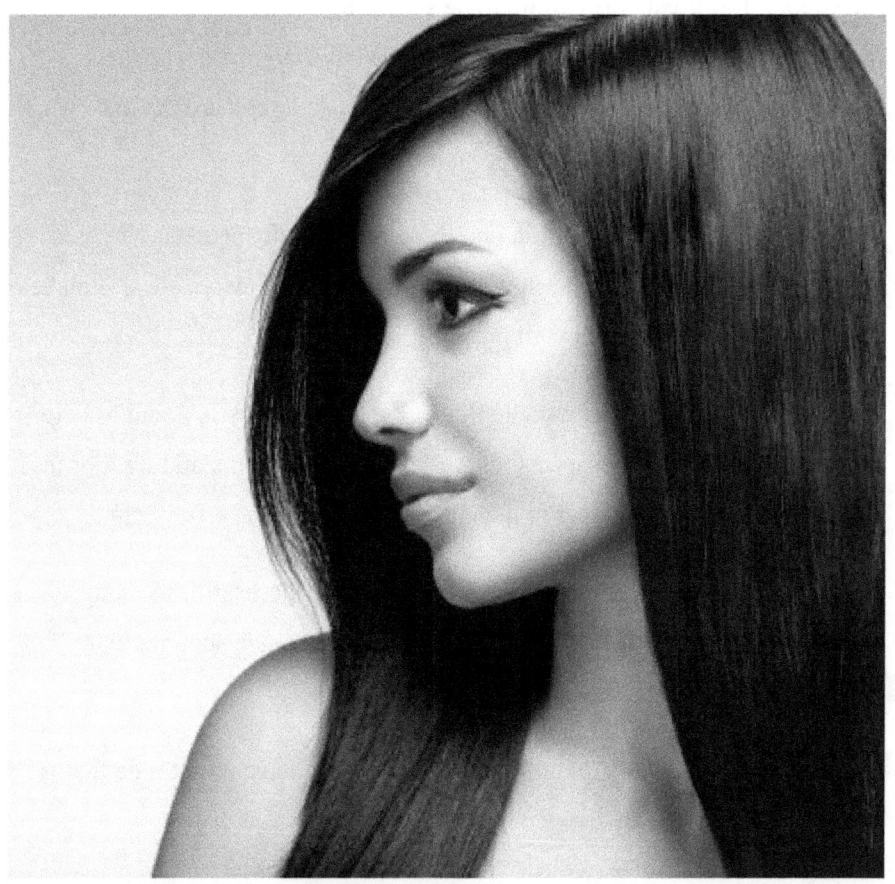

Why I am telling you this is because I know of a number of people who have ruined a perfectly good face, because they wanted some alternations done, and that according to them, would make them feel really beautiful, happy, and content. And then, I saw them looking at the mirror, happy with the result – for all of two minutes. After that, they wanted something else altered. That would really make them feel really happy…

Now for such a person, I can only say that even if they are molded in perfection, they are always going to be searching for that elusive chimera of what they do not have and what they want. Want shall always be their master, and they are never going to be satisfied. And they are the ones who make cosmetic surgeons multimillionaires.

But, as I say, if you can afford it, and there is no medical reason why you cannot have cosmetic surgery done, if you want it, and also well, if it makes you feel happy and secure by all means!

In many parts of the world, people think cosmetic surgery is going to help them in their marriage prospects, as well as in their social standing. For that, I can only say that it is going to depend upon one's own self-esteem.

If beauty were the only criteria to keep a marriage successful, so many beautiful people of Hollywood would not have had made such regular wrecks of their marriages than ever so often.

It is the change in your psychological makeup and personal attitude that is going to make all the difference in the long run.

An attractive outer exterior is helpful and beneficial, but not hundred percent successful for social and marital success.

When I was talking about this aspect, with my cosmetic surgeon friend, he told me that a number of people came to him for plastic surgery and he told them that they had skin diseases or inactive thyroid problems. That was the reason why the skin had started sagging. If they had gone straight to their GP, they would have been cured by now!

So, before you go in for any type of cosmetic surgical procedure, would not you want to get a full checkup done?

Facelifts

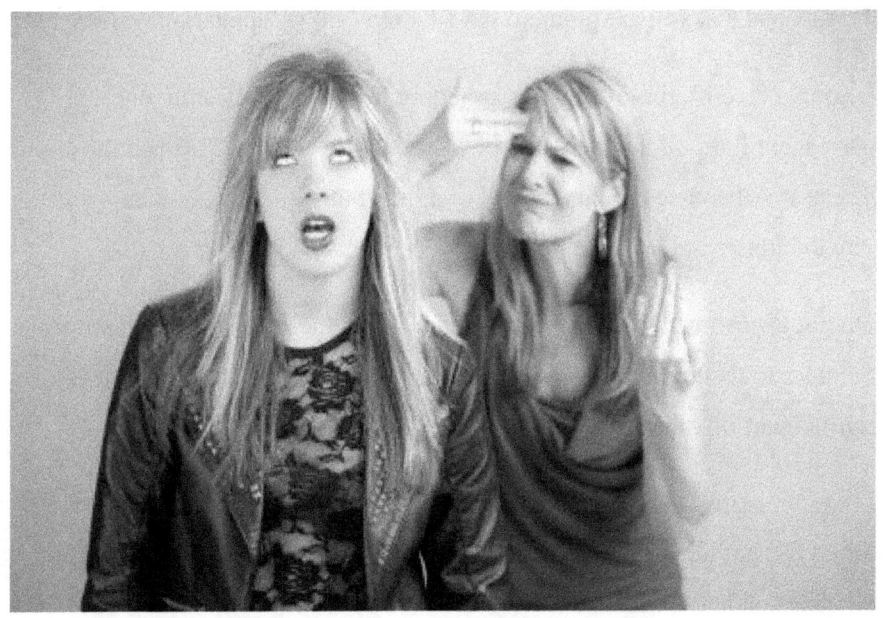

What is the matter with you? You want a facelift at your age?

Now just imagine you are a complete layman, and you want to know about facelifts. What do they mean?

Like I said before wrinkles are a normal part of the daily wear and tear of life. As you grow older, the tissues of your body are going to lose its elasticity. This process is going to be speeded if you have zero fat content. If you do not have fat in your body, how is your skin going to look plump, elastic and youthful?

Also, imagine, for instance, you have had the added misfortune of losing your teeth at an early age. The shape of your face is now totally changed, with the bones of the face, trying to adapt themselves to the new dentures. This means that you are going to have more wrinkles appearing and sooner.

During a facelift, these surgeons are going to get rid of a number of the permanent lines on the face, the folds around the neck, and around the jaws. These are of course part and parcel of aging, but getting rid of them gives you the illusion of youthfulness.

Do not expect them to remove the crease fold which is going to extend from the nose to the tip of your mouth. This is impossible to remove and it is a normal part of your facial tissue.

I remember my mother looking at me very carefully, about three decades ago. I did not have a crease fold. She had it, by the age of 13. She also had wrinkles on her forehead.

I would not know the reasons for those crease folds and those wrinkles at such a young age, but a teenager in the 50s would definitely not think about any sort of cosmetic surgery in order to get rid of the wrinkles and even those deep slashes/creases on one's face.

But today, I was astonished when a little girl of 10 went into depression because her mother did not want her to undergo plastic surgery so that she could have a snub nose like Walt Disney's Tinkerbell!

This dangerous trend is definitely disturbing, especially when the media is encouraging children to be more beauty conscious, in keeping with gender stereotypes, especially that nasty little perfect little Barbie doll.

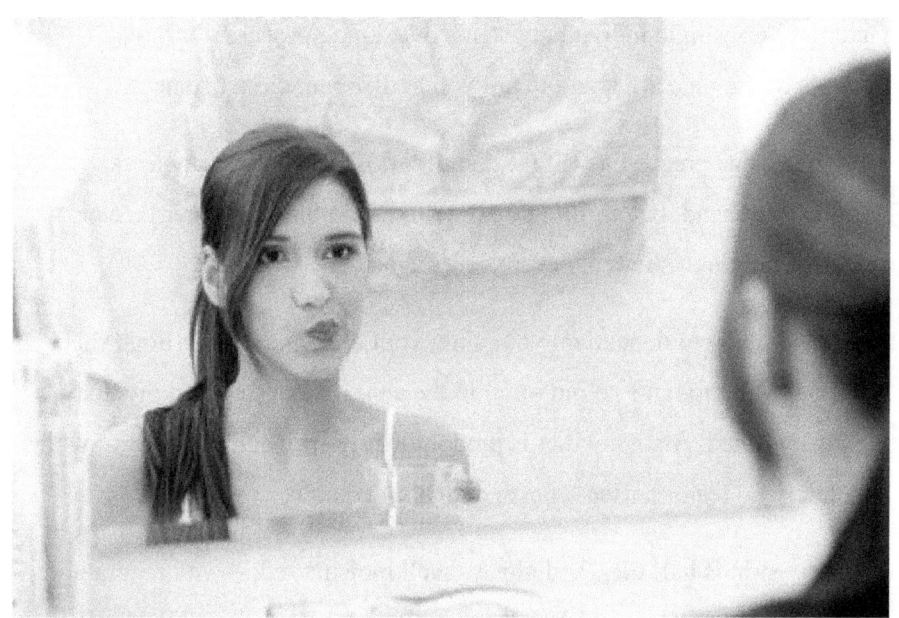

Is that a wrinkle I see?

Nevertheless, a facelift is going to please you, because you are going to think that you have managed to gain a more youthful appearance, notwithstanding the scars. Anybody who has a facelift operation is ready to go back to work within two – four weeks, depending on the bruises and scars which occur during the procedure.

Bruises, you say? Of course there is going to be a discoloration in that particular area because the surgeon has done some removal of tissue, and even though he may be very experienced and careful, he is going to leave some vestiges of activity, having been done in that particular area.

Even though the term is called a facelift in popular jargon, surgeons are going to call it surgery for the aging face. This is going to depend on many factors. Every single individual has his own aging process. Different portions of the face are going to aid you to different circumstances.

My mother had crease lines at the age of 13. Her daughter may have a wrinkled forehead, but absolutely no wrinkles on the rest of her face or body, even though she will never see 45 again.

All this is going to depend on your skin, your diet, and also through sheer luck! So even though I go out often in the sun, I make sure that my body is well dehydrated. Also, my diet is predominantly fruit and vegetables, with absolutely no tea or coffee – never caught that habit.

Also, my skin is half oily, and always well moisturized, – with natural oils and absolutely no chemical-based cosmetics – which means that it is not going to wrinkle so easily.

That means I will never have to undergo a facelift ever, not that I want to. This is one factor which the doctor is going to take into account. He is going to see how prone your face is to wrinkles and also the texture and elasticity of the skin

If it is as wrinkled as a walnut, and you have this bad habit of going out in the sun again, and again, well, however many facelifts, you get done, they are going to be wrinkles appearing at different places.

Also a number of ladies who are prone to crash diets are going to suffer from wrinkles. Just imagine that you had a nice plump face. And then somebody suggested a crash diet, and for the next three months or so you survived on a meager diet.

.

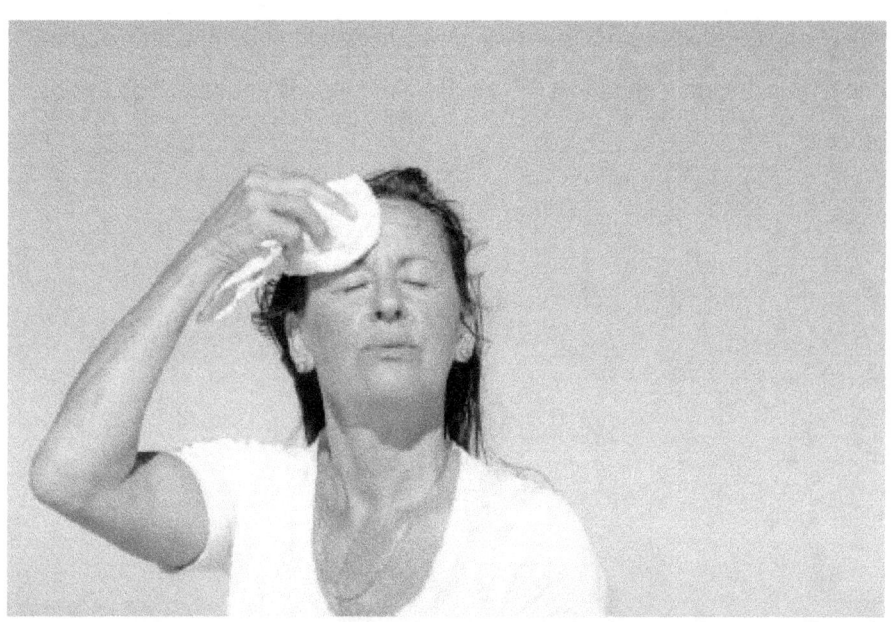

Dehydrated skin is going to cause more of wrinkles and faster...

So all right, you lost weight. But look at your face. The body, which is in salvation survival mode, has taken the fat from the fatty tissue in your face, to keep your system working properly. You do not know that fat is necessary for keeping the body functioning in a healthy manner. You want to get rid of it.

But your body in survival mode is using the fatty layers present in the body tissue, because not only is your body, not having the necessary nutrients needed to keep your body healthy, but you are on a zero fat diet.

So your nice plump face is now a haggard, wrinkled face, because its underlying tissue of fat has been expended in keeping you alive.

Also, you are going to find the skin on the neck and under the jaw sagging, due to this drastic weight loss. Naturally, your skin is going to look terribly older.

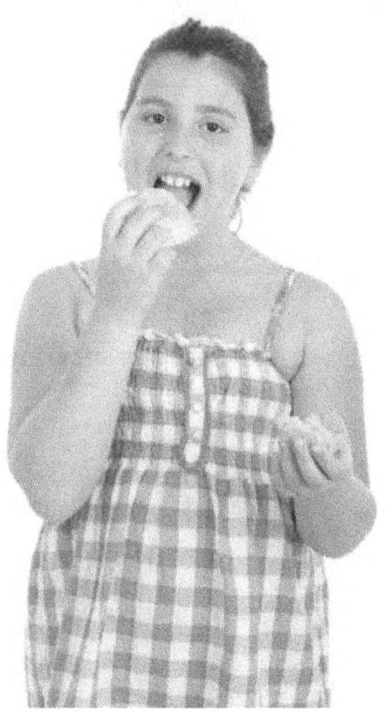

If she ever goes on a diet, the first visible effect is going to be seen on her face.

So the moment you go on a diet, your face is going to show the visible effects. First the skin is going to sag, and then you are going to see wrinkles appearing.

That is why, my advice is that if you are planning on a facelift, lose weight first. Reach your goals of desired poundage. After that, go in for a cosmetic surgery procedure.

After the surgery has been done, you can put on some more weight, if you wish, and fill in your face if you wish.

Deep Wrinkle Removal

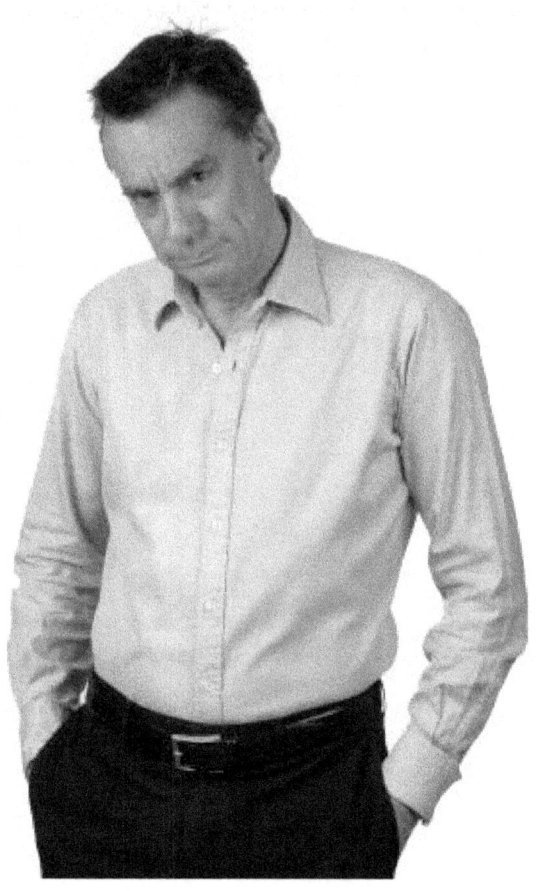

What do you mean, I have wrinkles on my forehead?

Just wrinkle up your forehead. Oh, my where did those deep wrinkles come from? I remember asking an old lady this, and the tender age of seven, frowning away in her antique mirror. And she answered me with a very nice ancient story, about How the Lord of Creation used to visit every newborn child at night, and write his fate with his iron pen upon his forehead. Once those lines were drawn, nobody could change them.

So everybody had those lines embedded deep in the forehead.

This is an interesting myth, but it is a well-known fact that many of us have deep issues about the lines on our forehead. So how do you get about getting rid of them?

Remember that if you keep persisting on frowning, these lines are going to get even more prominent and apparent. A forehead with wrinkles, presents a great problem for cosmetic surgeons, because they have to make an incision in the hairline, depending on the nature of the wrinkles.

These incisions are going to be either on each side or on the top of the scalp. This procedure is to elevate the forehead through a front temporal approach.

That means that they are going to take the forehead right down to the eyebrows and then divide the portion of the muscles that cause the wrinkles. Gadzooks! However, cosmetic surgeons try their best to make sure that the patient has a scar high in the forehead, which can be hidden by the hairline.

And that is why this is not the sort of operation that can be done to any patient. The muscular tissue in that particular area is going to be weakened, and there is sometimes a temporary numbness of the skull and of the earlobes.

But people are prepared to pay the price of this sort of discomfiture for the sake of beauty, vanity and a smooth forehead.

That is why I would rather have my wrinkled forehead.

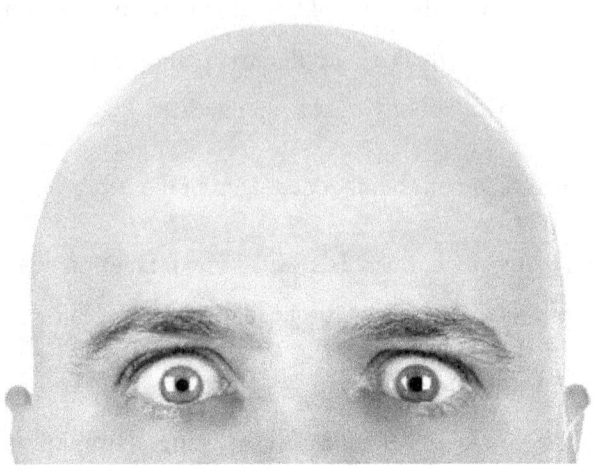

Look, no lines on my forehead at all! Or anywhere else for that matter!

Now let us come to eyelid surgery and crows – feet removal.

Eyelid Surgery and Crows – Feet Removal

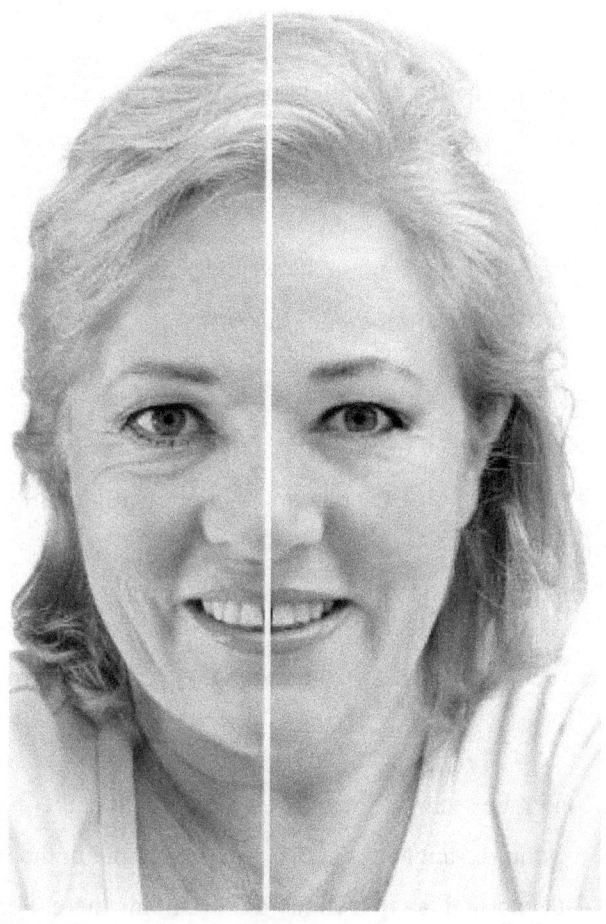

Eyelid surgery definitely comes in the very delicate operational procedure and it is approached with great care by experienced surgeons. In fact, any sort of eye surgery is going to be treated with great delicacy and should be undertaken by an experienced cosmetic surgeon.

Everybody knows that the eyes show the aging process of the face, more easily. Tired eyes are going to make you look older, but most of the time, the pouches and the bags and the wrinkles around your eyes mean that you have had too many late night parties in smoke filled atmospheres.

And also you have not had your eight hours of your necessary beauty sleep. The pollution ridden atmosphere of the city also ages your skin around your eyes prematurely.

Now, when a surgeon operates upon the wrinkles around the eyes, he has to take into account the excessive amount of skin on the upper and lower eyelids.

Sometimes it is the presence of excessive fatty tissue, which makes your skin look baggy. This is going to show most prominently in the corners, near the nose and mainly in the upper eyelids.

On the other hand, crows – feet is because the whole face is aging. What surgeons do in such cases is that they remove the excess skin from the upper eyelid.

The incision cannot be seen with your eyes open and then the incision is extended out beyond the angle of the eye. The scar is put in the line of the crows – feet – it is normal for everybody to have a line there. For the corner of the eyelids, the surgeon has to make sure that the incision is laced under the eyelashes.

Then the fat is removed, both from the upper and lower. I did.

If you have a great problem of crows – feet, you cannot solve it with just eyelid reduction. They are going to extend all out on to the face.

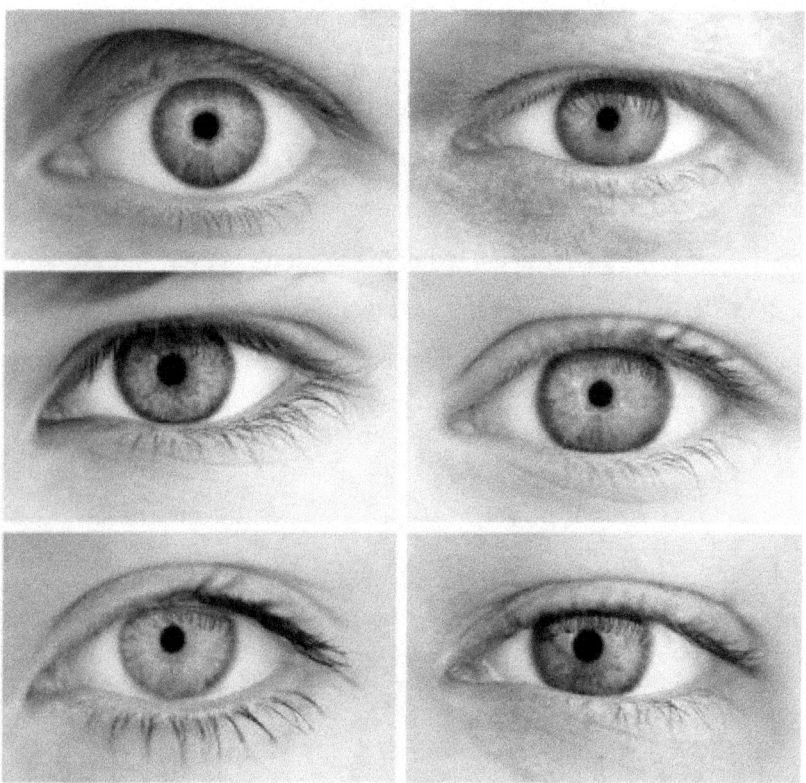

That is where you may be advised to go in for the Temple pull. In this procedure, the surgeon is going to pull the skin from the temple region. However, many experienced surgeons suggest that it is better to have a facelift done, first, and any eyelid treatment done afterwards.

Nose and Neck Surgery

Rhinoplasty, nose surgery, is one of the most popular of cosmetic procedures. This is when the surgeon is going to remodel the tip of the nose after breaking it. Sometimes they do an incision to help with the breathing process. That is because you are going to have a plaster on your nose for 10 – 12 days. That also means for the next two weeks you are going to be out of the count, socially, and only your near and dear ones are going to know that you are getting a "nose procedure" done to your own satisfaction.

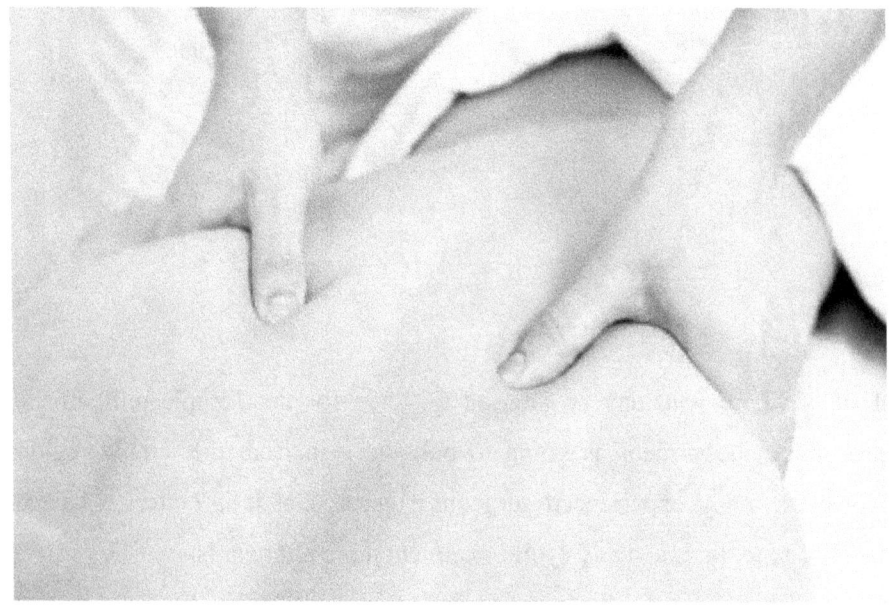

You can get rid of some of the fat with massage.

The neck can either be thick or as scrawny as a chicken neck. What he is surgeon is going to do is she is going to pull the neck skin up to the face.

This excess facial skin is going to go behind the ears. It is then going to be removed. The marks are thus going to be found behind the ears.

But what if you have an extremely thin neck or a really fat neck? The fat is going to be removed during the surgical procedure. But sometimes it is the neck is too thin and there are too many wrinkles, the doctor is going to consider making an incision under the skin and pulling up the skin from there

What they might not tell you beforehand is that they cannot remove scars. They can just improve the appearance of scars. Scars are inevitable.

In the same manner, if you have wrinkles around the mouth, cosmetic surgeons do not remove them by facelifts. They suggest a procedure called dermabrasion, which is going to mean the removal of the first layer of the skin. The only problem is that skin color around the mouth is going to look different from the normal skin texture and tone.

Breast Surgery

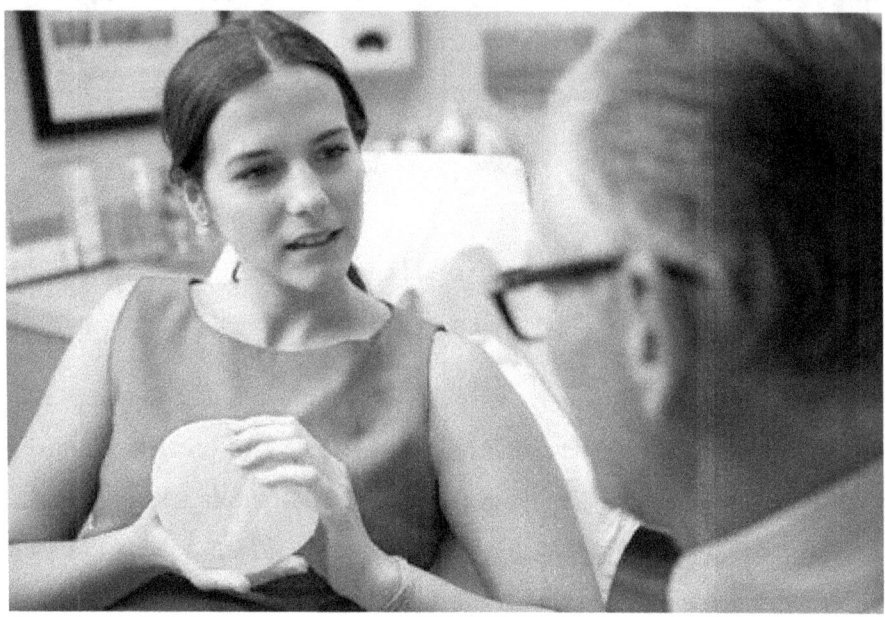

A number of women go in for this particular surgical procedure because they are under the impression that this improves the shape of the breasts and make them look like the popular version and concept of Mother Goddess.

My cosmetic surgeon friend told me that this is another procedure, which has him singing all the way to the bank. But he also told me that many women do not know that they are different sizes of breasts. If genetically they have inherited small breasts, they cannot just show their favorite cosmetic surgeon, a photograph of 42 – 24 – 36 and request them to make them look like a Coca-Cola bottle or Jayne Mansfield.

So that is the reason why the surgeons always make sure that they meet the patient's desire, according to their other features. The real practical ones may not understand why women want to go around with enormous busts because they know all about how lopsided the center of gravity of such a misshapen person can be, taking into account the size.

But as a practical advisor, take me tell you something. Such a huge bosom may gain you brownie points with the audience, especially if you associate popularity with the size of your bra, but you are definitely going to suffer from bra rashes because of inadequate support. Also, you are going to sweat profusely.

Let me give you a practical example in my own family. Many of the ladies on the maternal side are prone to be "tiny" – between 5' 4" and 5' 6". And all of them have genetically inherited size 44-46 bosoms.

I remember going to the ancestral maternal village as a child and looking at awe at all these ladies who were the epitome of Eastern beauty with the three B's – bosom, belly, and behind. And all of them complained in private that they were so uncomfortable with that extra weight everywhere.

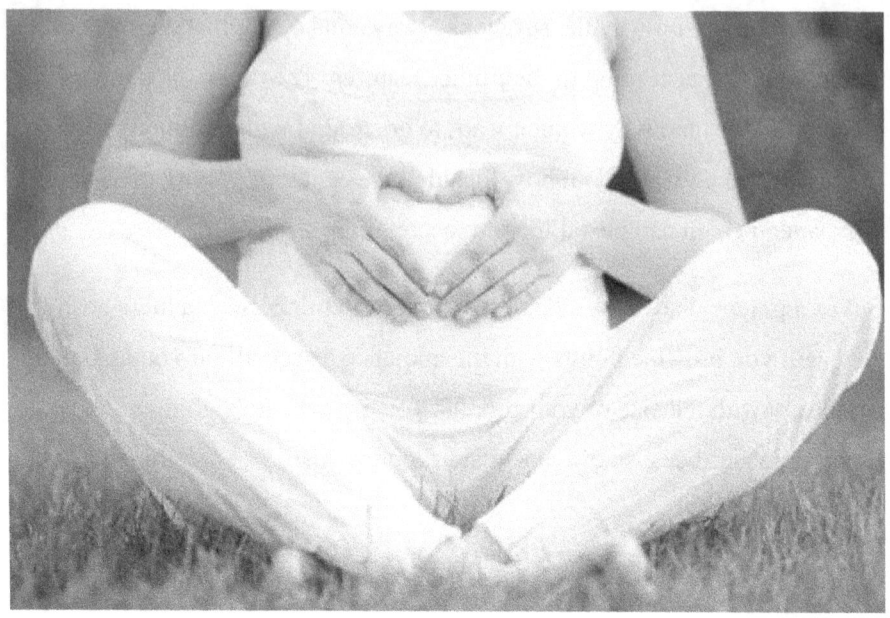

However, their mindset is that such a woman is desirable, because she is supposedly "healthy" enough to bear many, many children. And so they took it for granted that a heavy bosom, lots of belly, and behind was related to being 110% female .[3]

This concept is also accepted in many parts of the West, especially in Europe – namely Spain, Italy and the Nordic countries.

---

[3] Thankfully I managed to escape this onerous burden due to my father's stronger lean and thin gene line. But my maternal relatives have managed to entertain themselves down the years, by just taking one look at me and asking if I got enough of food to eat, because I was as skinny as a skeleton, and definitely not their idea of a beautiful desirable female and a future fecund earth mother! Again, as I said before, Pfui!

What many of the ladies with heavy busts do not know that the alignment of the shoulder is going to get disturbed as they are pulled forward due to excess weight in the upper portion of their torso.

That is why it is much more preferable and sensible to have small or medium-sized breasts. However, social trends , and masculine mindsets make females want to believe that huge enormous breasts are what men prefer, and females keep trying to live up to that particular ancient and deep-rooted concept of feminine beauty.[4]

There are different methods normally followed by surgeons like putting on a breast prosthesis, which goes under a small breast to make it look larger. Or living skin is used to shape the breast. New methods and surgical procedures are appearing every day, as the future of cosmetic surgery expands even more.

---

[4] That reminds me of one of Jayne Mansfield's wartime efforts, Kiss the Boys for Me, in which she is this nitwit squealing and giggling away on the dance floor with a soldier on leave. A woman tags her with these words "38." And JM responds with a triumphant "40 "and continues propelling her partner around the dance floor. So this is supposed to tell the audience that one can have an IQ of a boiled rutabaga, but if the bust size is 40, that dame is going to get all the guys. Does not say much about the IQ level of the men either!

Liposuction and Tummy tucks

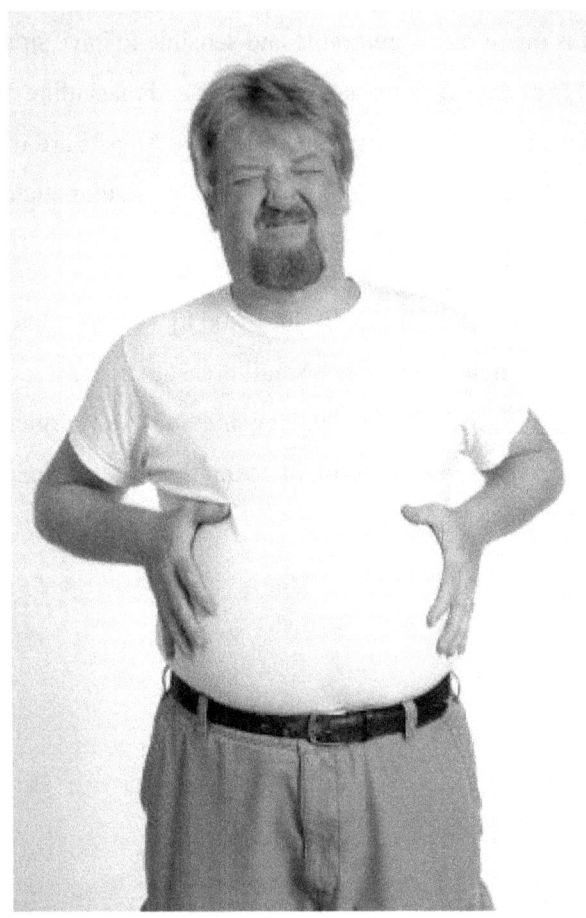

Liposuction is the removal of fatty tissue from under the epidermis.
Different surgical procedures are used to get rid of this fat, especially around
the thighs, hips, or any region where there is a fatty deposit.

The problem of stomach tucks can be divided in two parts. One is normally going to show up as stretch marks, which are associated with pregnancy and are due to the normal hormonal influence. This means that there is going to be excess of skin on the stomach region, but some women can get them on the thighs, breasts and posterior region depending on the hormone quantity secreted.

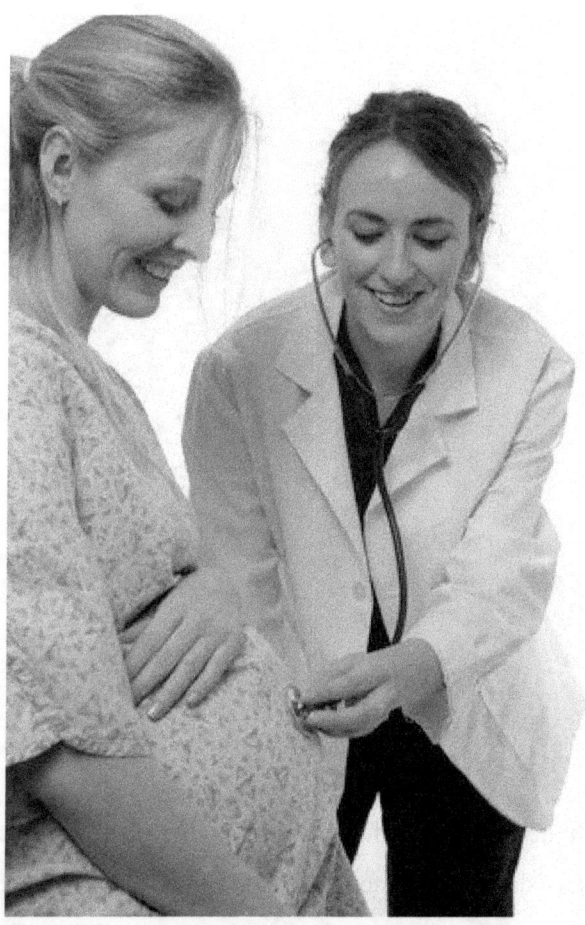

Stretch marks are a natural and normal side effect of pregnancy.

Stretch marks can also be due to weight loss, and the shrinkage of skin, especially in the abdominal muscles and region.

If one has lost weight, all of a sudden, the flabby muscles are going to appear. These muscles are just like overstretched elastic.

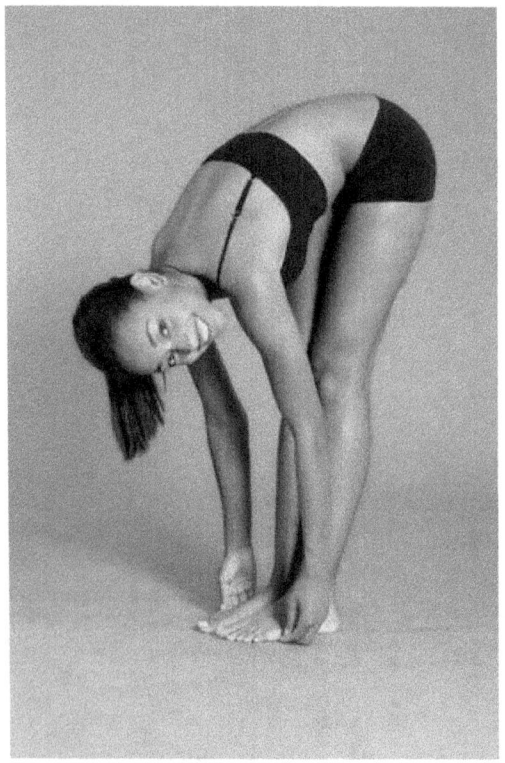

Surgeons normally make sure that any woman patient who wants to have cosmetic surgery done on the stomach region finishes having a family first. That is because another pregnancy is going to cancel all the effects of the surgery.

For fat people who find they have plenty of extra skin showing thanks to losing weight, the surgeons just cut off that extra skin and sew the tissue, but sometimes when the patient is still overweight and wants the surgeons took got off the excess fat, they are told to go on a proper and sensibly controlled diet, which is going to be more beneficial.

After that they are going to be helped with stomach tucks.

Fat bottoms and thighs are not a matter of obesity alone. Many times you are going to find that the top region of the torso is slim, but the lower region can be considered to be "solid and fatty." This is possibility genetic and an inherited trait.

Exercise can reduce the fat there and then the extra skin can be cut off by an experienced cosmetic surgeon.

Conclusion

This book has given you plenty of information about cosmetic surgery, and if you really need it.

If you are going in for any sort of surgical procedure, including cosmetic surgery, you may want to take the advice of the surgeon who is going to take in view, the reason for the surgery, the psychological factor governing this decision, the state of the health of the patient and other factors.

Remember that like every surgical procedure, cosmetic surgery can also cause infections, especially when they are done by unqualified surgeons. So make sure that if you are going in for such a procedure, you ask around first from happy patients, who tell you all about the success rate, the post-operational care, the charges, and other tips pertaining to that particular surgeon, his experience, his skills and his efficacy.

Naturally you are going to be seeing the visible effects of his handwork when you meet some of these patients face to face.

Live Long and Prosper!

Author Bio

Dueep Jyot Singh is a Management and IT Professional who managed to gather Postgraduate qualifications in Management and English and Degrees in Science, French and Education while pursuing different enjoyable career options like being an hospital administrator, IT,SEO and HRD Database Manager/ trainer, movie , radio and TV scriptwriter, theatre artiste and public speaker, lecturer in French, Marketing and Advertising, ex-Editor of Hearts On Fire (now known as Solstice) Books Missouri USA, advice columnist and cartoonist, publisher and Aviation School trainer, ex-moderator on Medico.in, banker, student councilor ,travelogue writer … among other things!

One fine morning, she decided that she had enough of killing herself by Degrees and went back to her first love -- writing. It's more enjoyable! She already has 48 published academic and 14 fiction- in- different- genre books under her belt.

When she is not designing websites or making Graphic design illustrations for clients , she is browsing through old bookshops hunting for treasures, of which she has an enviable collection – including R.L. Stevenson, O.Henry, Dornford Yates, Maurice Walsh, De Maupassant, Victor Hugo, Sapper, C.N. Williamson, "Bartimeus" and the crown of her collection- Dickens "The Old Curiosity Shop," and "Martin Chuzzlewit" and so on… Just call her "Renaissance Woman") - collecting herbal remedies, acting like Universal Helping Hand/Agony Aunt, or escaping to her dear mountains for a bit of exploring, collecting herbs and plants and trekking.

Check out some of the other JD-Biz Publishing books

Gardening Series on Amazon

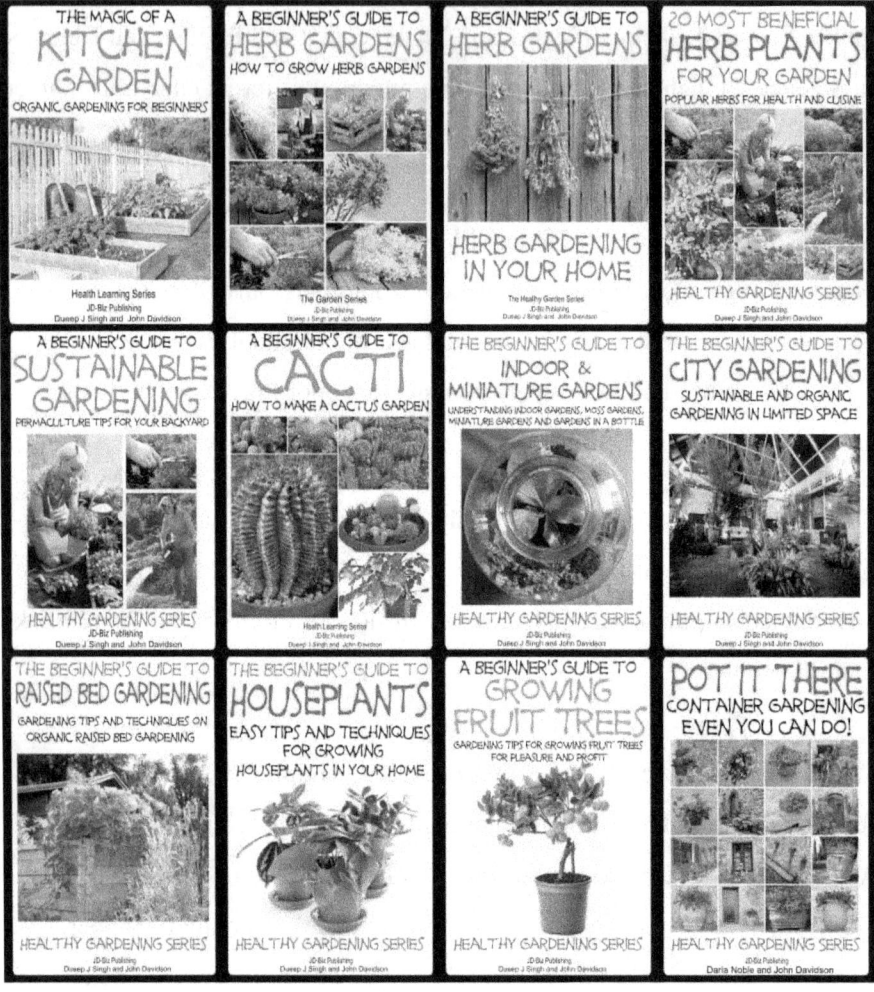

Health Learning Series

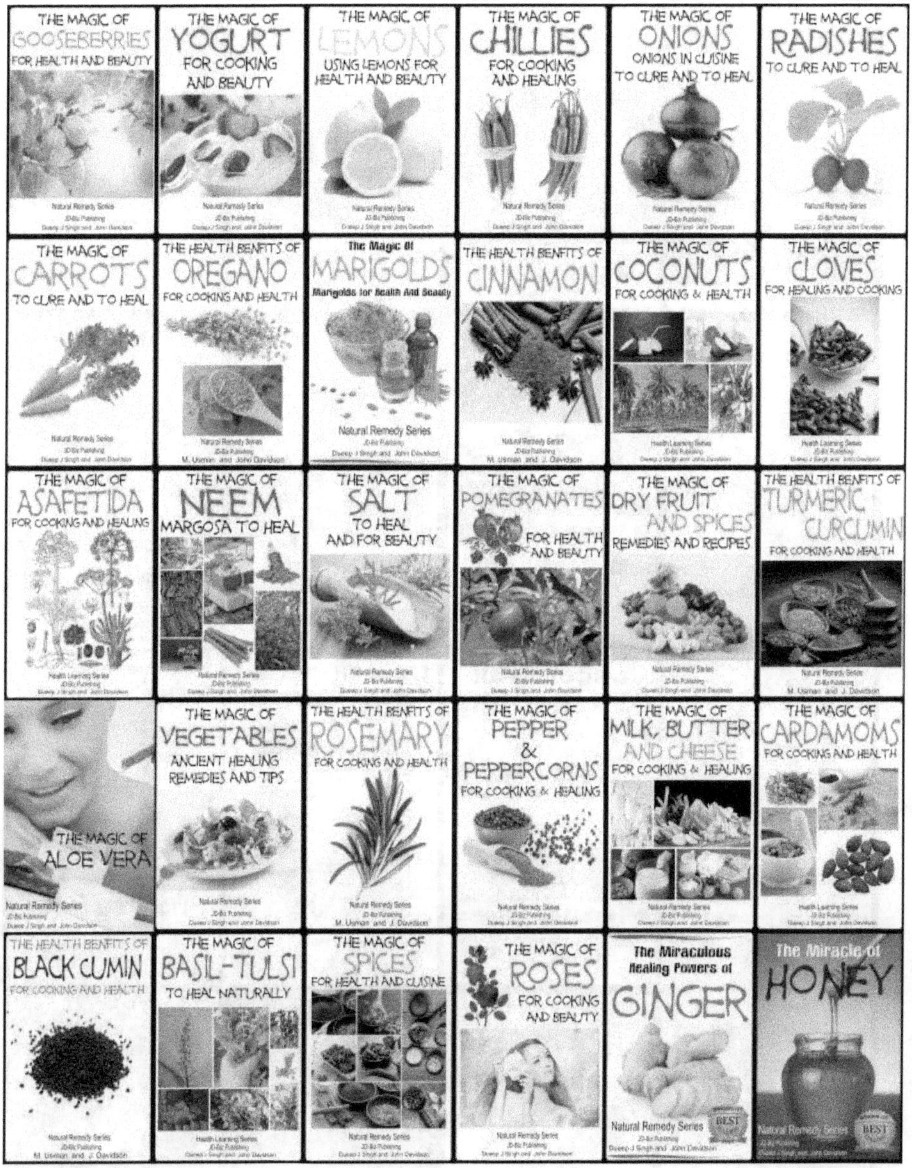

Country Life Books

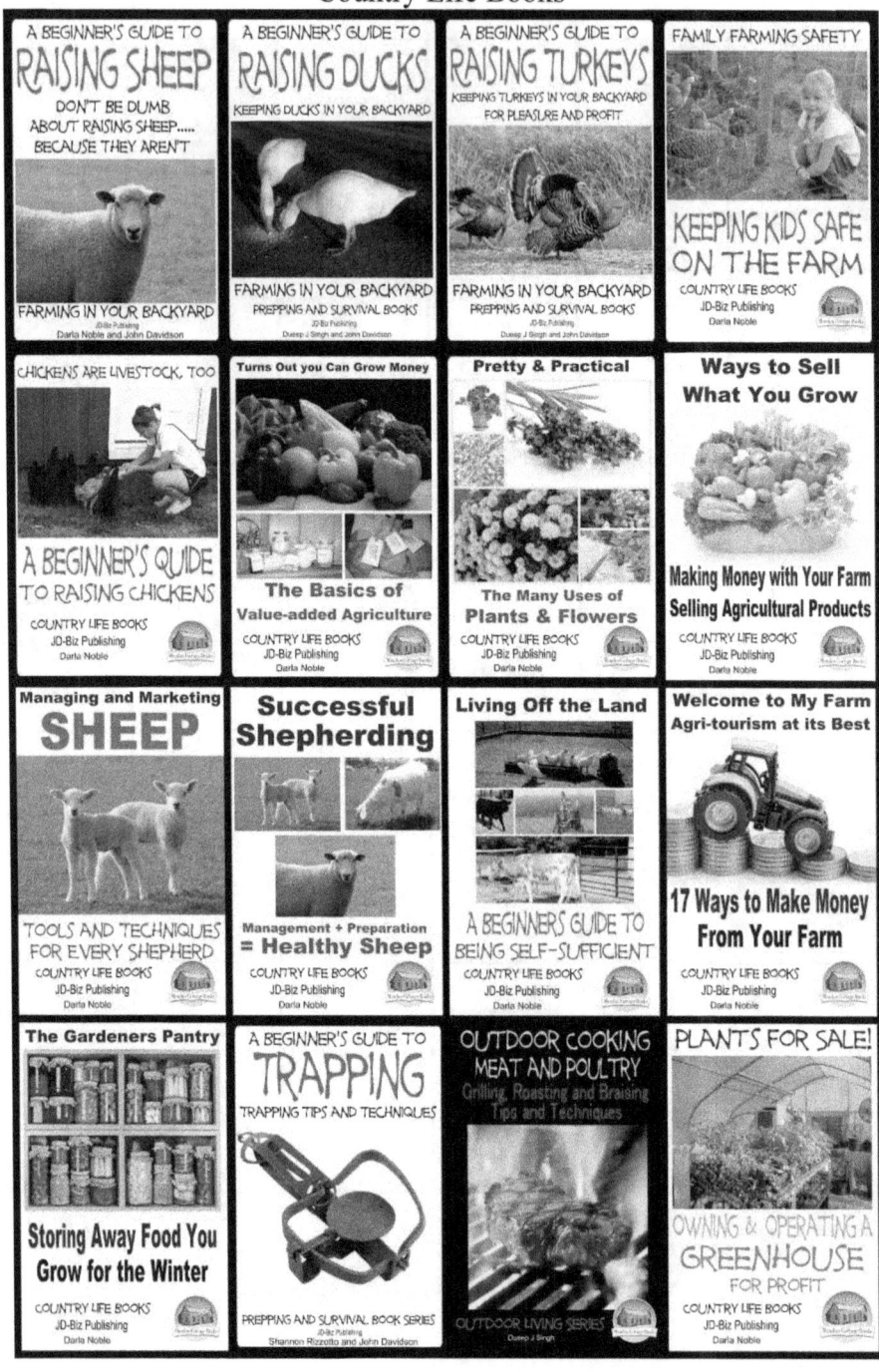

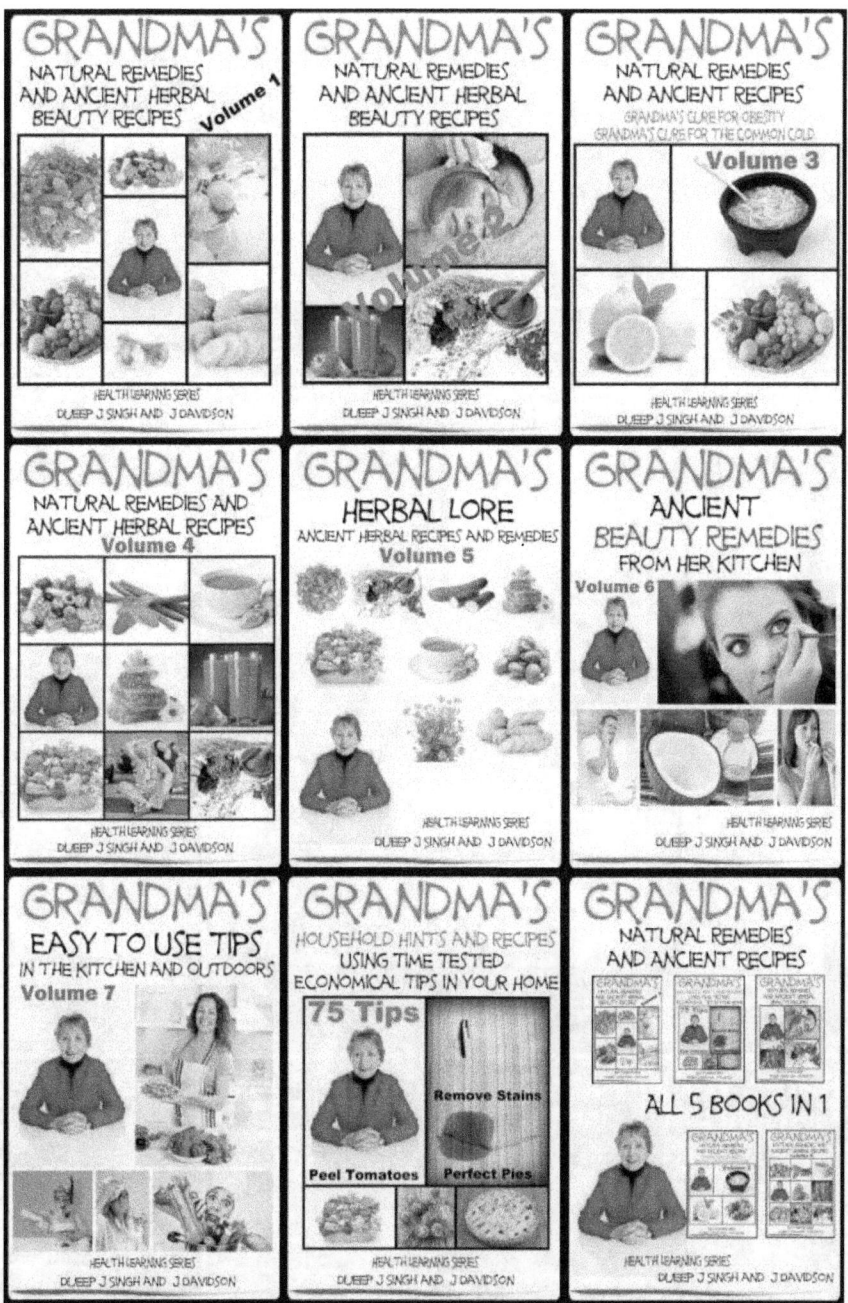

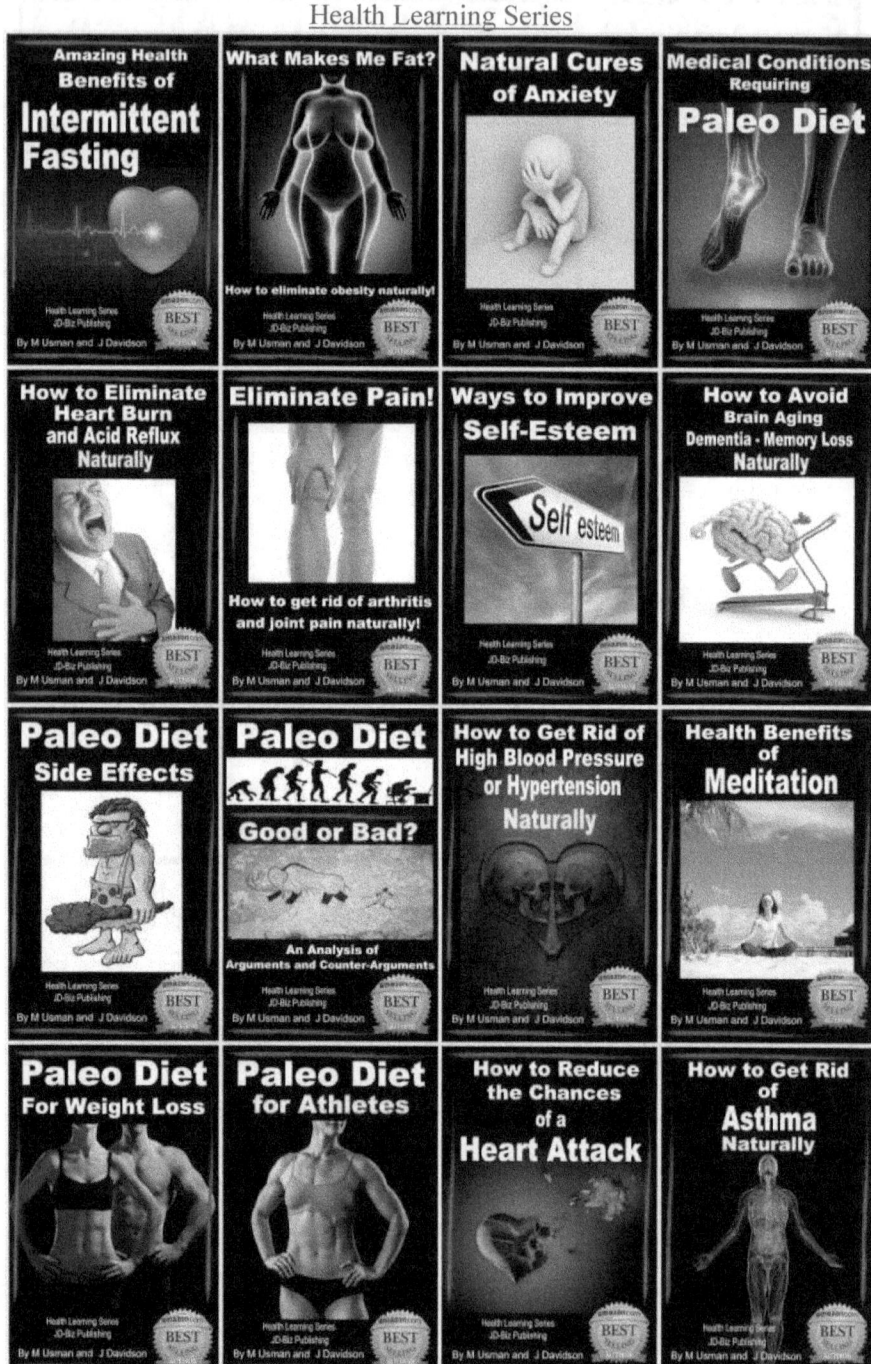

Amazing Animal Book Series

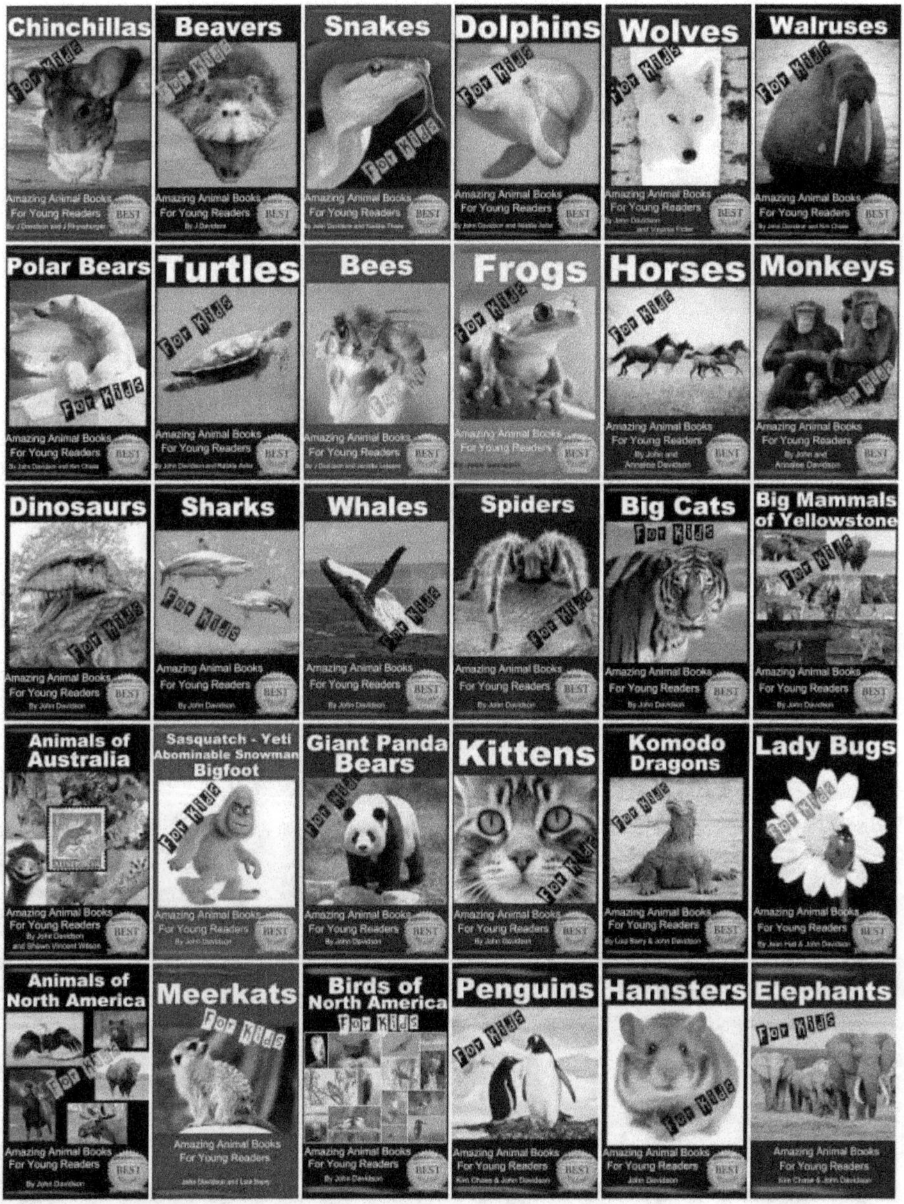

Learn To Draw Series

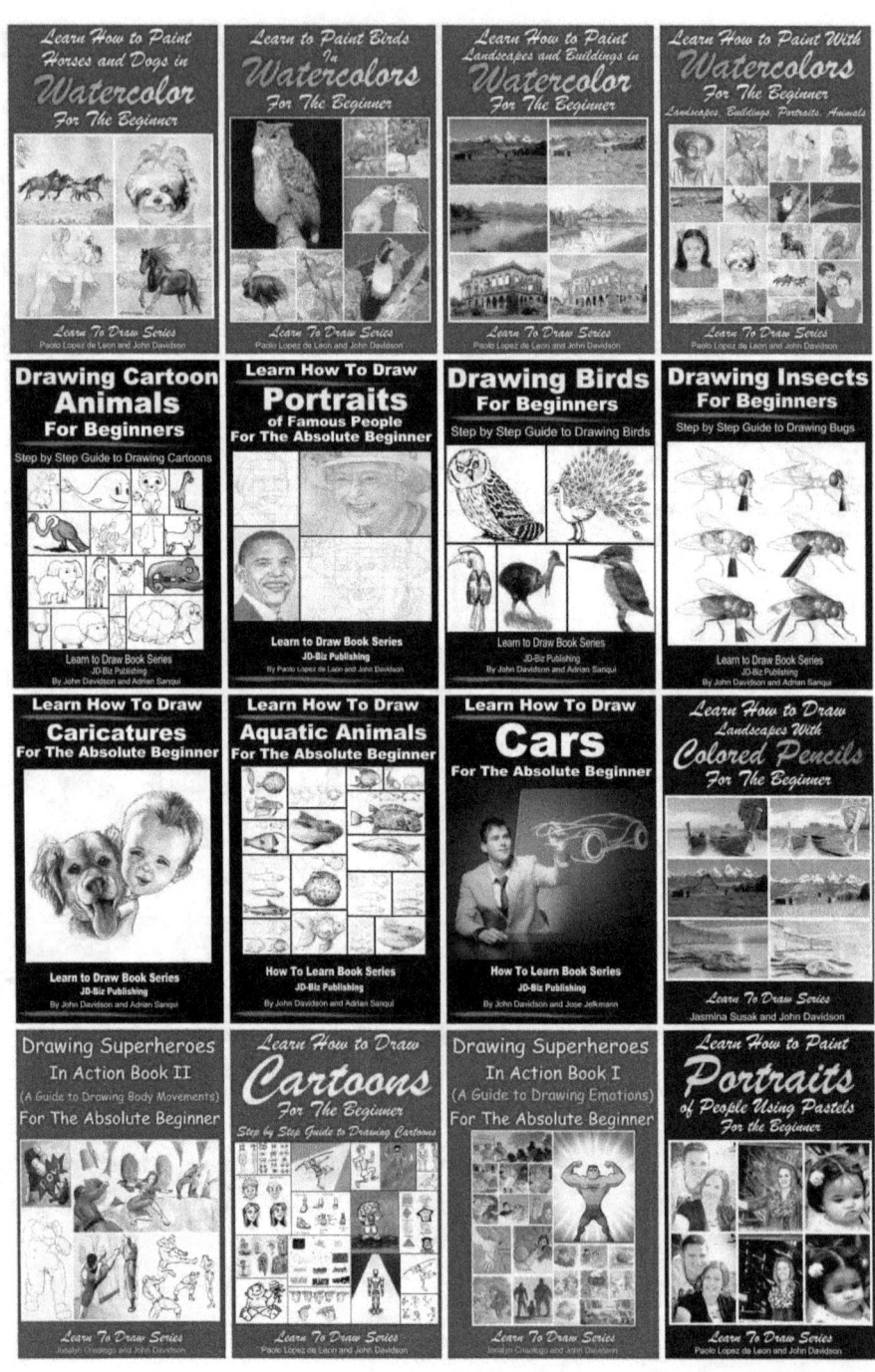

How to Build and Plan Books

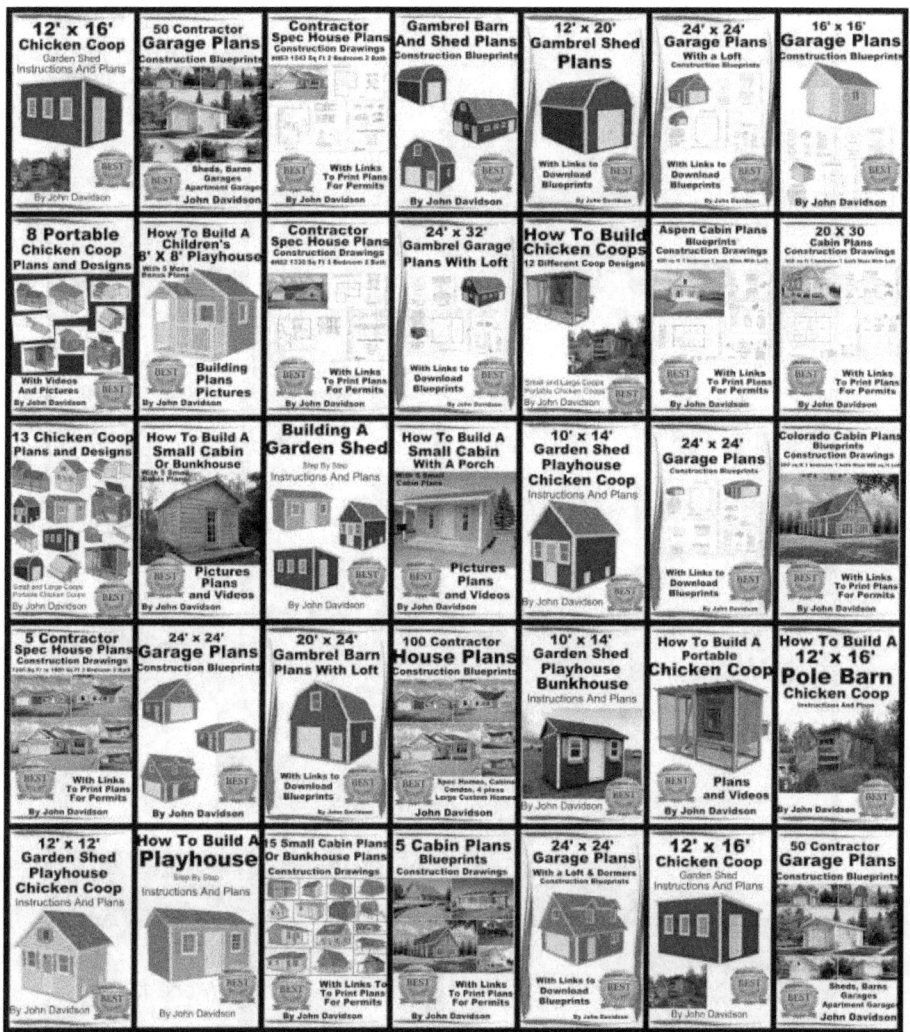

Entrepreneur Book Series

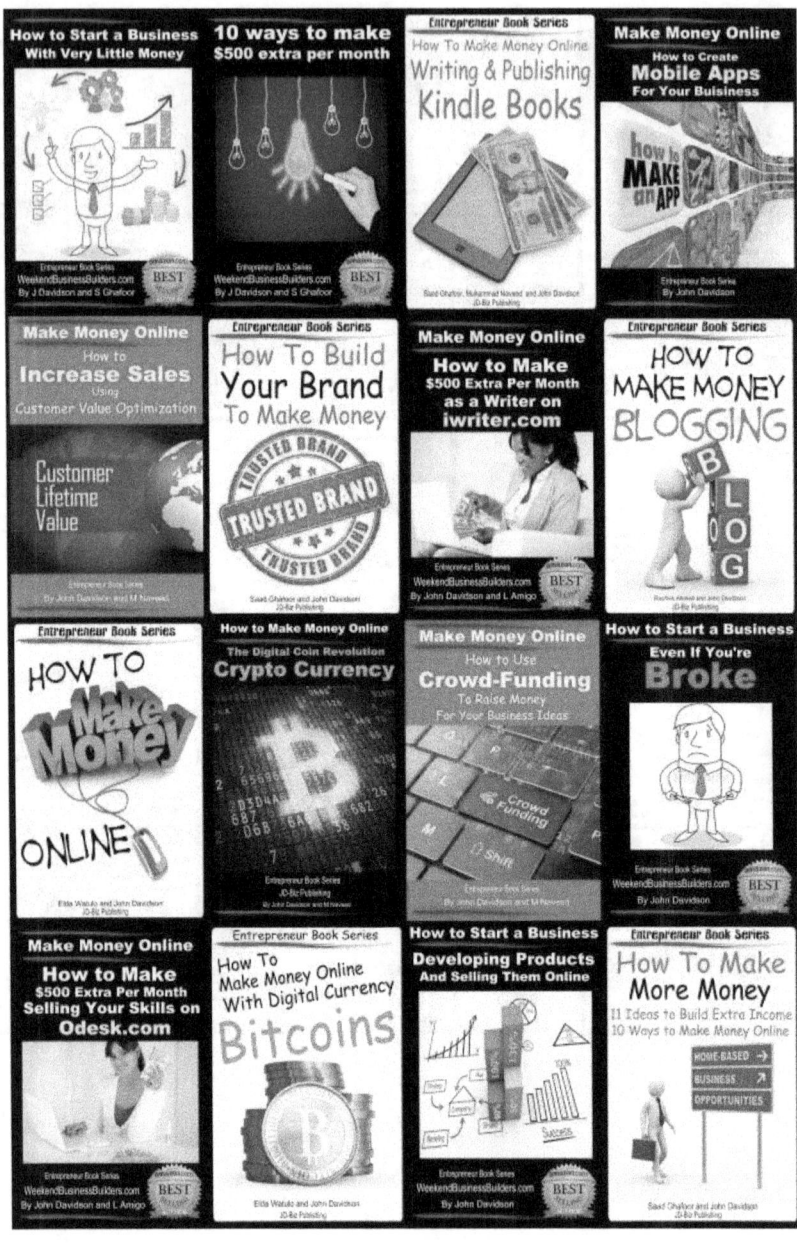

Our books are available at

1. Amazon.com

2. Barnes and Noble

3. Itunes

4. Kobo

5. Smashwords

6. Google Play Books

Publisher

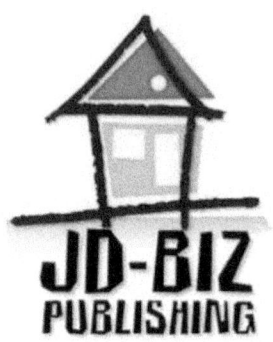

JD-Biz Corp

P O Box 374

Mendon, Utah 84325

http://www.jd-biz.com/

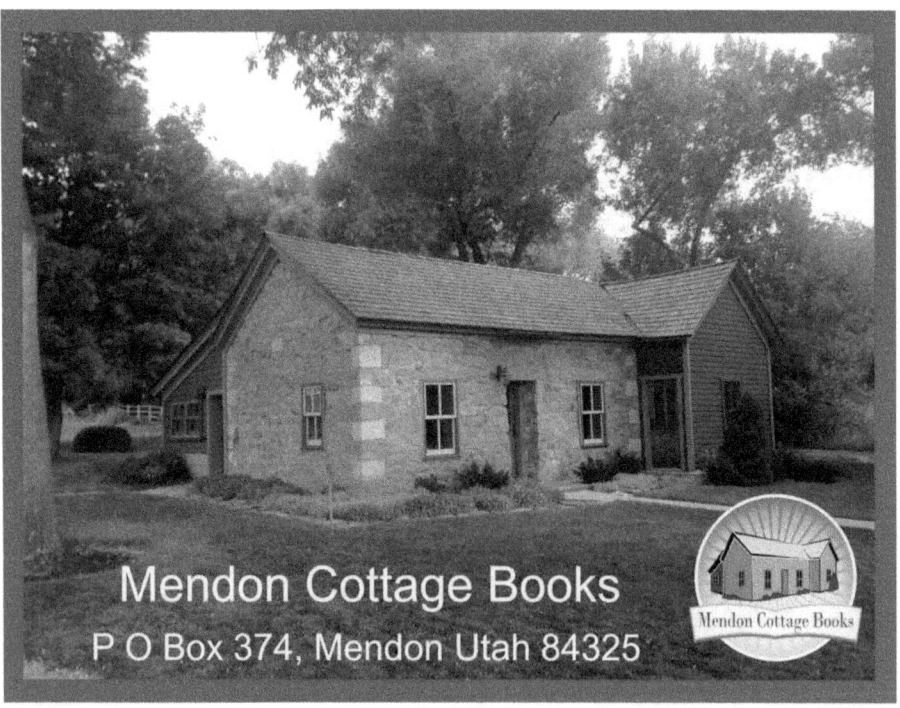